This journal belongs to:
_____

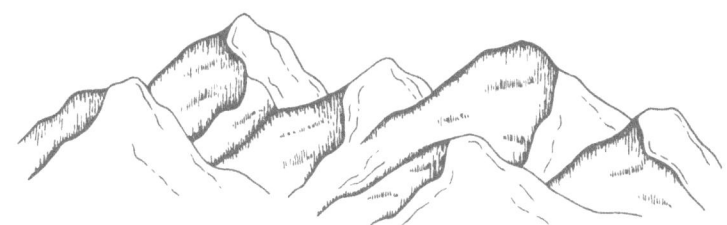

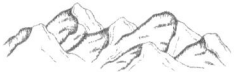

Date:_____

"Every day presents an opportunity to try something new or to move something one step closer to completion."

Date:_____

"Every day presents an opportunity to try something new or to move something one step closer to completion."

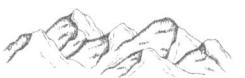

Date:_____

"Every day presents an opportunity to try something new or to move something one step closer to completion."

Date:_____

"Every day presents an opportunity to try something new or to move something one step closer to completion."

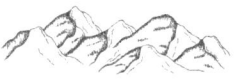

Date:_____

"Every day presents an opportunity to try something new or to move something one step closer to completion."

Date:_____

"Every day presents an opportunity to try something new or to move something one step closer to completion."

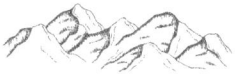

Date:_____

"Every day presents an opportunity to try something new or to move something one step closer to completion."

Date:_____

"Every day presents an opportunity to try something new or to move something one step closer to completion."

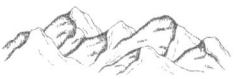

Date:_____

"Every day presents an opportunity to try something new or to move something one step closer to completion."

Date:_____

"Every day presents an opportunity to try something new or to move something one step closer to completion."

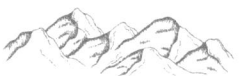

Date:_____

"Every day presents an opportunity to try something new or to move something one step closer to completion."

Date:_____

"Every day presents an opportunity to try something new or to move something one step closer to completion."

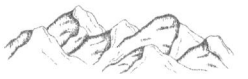

Date:_____

"Every day presents an opportunity to try something new or to move something one step closer to completion."

Date:_____

"Every day presents an opportunity to try something new or to move something one step closer to completion."

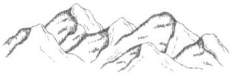

Date:_____

"Every day presents an opportunity to try something new or to move something one step closer to completion."

Date:_____

"Every day presents an opportunity to try something new or to move something one step closer to completion."

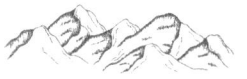

Date:_____

"Every day presents an opportunity to try something new or to move something one step closer to completion."

Date:_____

"Every day presents an opportunity to try something new or to move something one step closer to completion."

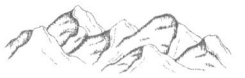

Date:_____

"Every day presents an opportunity to try something new or to move something one step closer to completion."

Date:_____

"Every day presents an opportunity to try something new or to move something one step closer to completion."

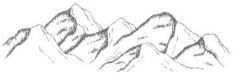

Date:_____

"Every day presents an opportunity to try something new or to move something one step closer to completion."

Date:_____

"Every day presents an opportunity to try something new or to move something one step closer to completion."

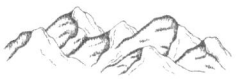

Date:_____

"Every day presents an opportunity to try something new or to move something one step closer to completion."

Date:_____

"Every day presents an opportunity to try something new or to move something one step closer to completion."

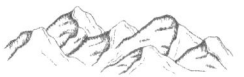

Date:_____

"Every day presents an opportunity to try something new or to move something one step closer to completion."

Date:_____

"Every day presents an opportunity to try something new or to move something one step closer to completion."

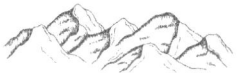

Date:_____

"Every day presents an opportunity to try something new or to move something one step closer to completion."

Date:_____

"Every day presents an opportunity to try something new or to move something one step closer to completion."

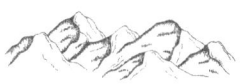

Date:_____

"Every day presents an opportunity to try something new or to move something one step closer to completion."

Date:_____

"Every day presents an opportunity to try something new or to move something one step closer to completion."

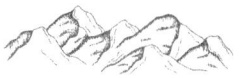

Date:_____

"Life is like a good meal. We know it's going to end sometime, so we have to savour every morsel."

Date:_____

"Life is like a good meal. We know it's going to end sometime, so we have to savour every morsel."

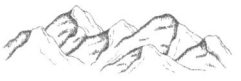

Date:_____

"Life is like a good meal. We know it's going to end sometime, so we have to savour every morsel."

Date:_____

"Life is like a good meal. We know it's going to end sometime, so we have to savour every morsel."

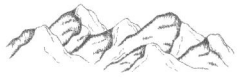

Date:_____

"Life is like a good meal. We know it's going to end sometime, so we have to savour every morsel."

Date:_____

"Life is like a good meal. We know it's going to end sometime, so we have to savour every morsel."

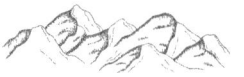

Date:_____

"Life is like a good meal. We know it's going to end sometime, so we have to savour every morsel."

Date:_____

"Life is like a good meal. We know it's going to end sometime, so we have to savour every morsel."

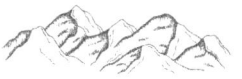

Date:_____

"Life is like a good meal. We know it's going to end sometime, so we have to savour every morsel."

Date:_____

"Life is like a good meal. We know it's going to end sometime, so we have to savour every morsel."

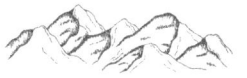

Date:_____

"Life is like a good meal. We know it's going to end sometime, so we have to savour every morsel."

Date:_____

"Life is like a good meal. We know it's going to end sometime, so we have to savour every morsel."

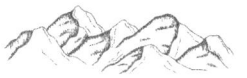

Date:_____

"Life is like a good meal. We know it's going to end sometime, so we have to savour every morsel."

Date:_____

"Life is like a good meal. We know it's going to end sometime, so we have to savour every morsel."

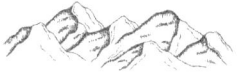

Date:_____

"Life is like a good meal. We know it's going to end sometime, so we have to savour every morsel."

Date:_____

"Life is like a good meal. We know it's going to end sometime, so we have to savour every morsel."

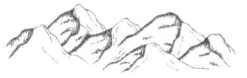

Date:_____

"Life is like a good meal. We know it's going to end sometime, so we have to savour every morsel."

Date:_____

"Life is like a good meal. We know it's going to end sometime, so we have to savour every morsel."

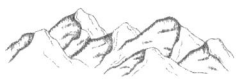

Date:_____

"Life is like a good meal. We know it's going to end sometime, so we have to savour every morsel."

Date:_____

"Life is like a good meal. We know it's going to end sometime, so we have to savour every morsel."

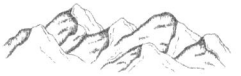

Date:_____

"Life is like a good meal. We know it's going to end sometime, so we have to savour every morsel."

Date:_____

"Life is like a good meal. We know it's going to end sometime, so we have to savour every morsel."

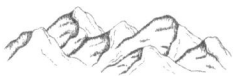

Date:_____

"Life is like a good meal. We know it's going to end sometime, so we have to savour every morsel."

Date:_____

"Life is like a good meal. We know it's going to end sometime, so we have to savour every morsel."

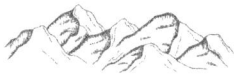

Date:_____

"Life is like a good meal. We know it's going to end sometime, so we have to savour every morsel."

Date:_____

"Life is like a good meal. We know it's going to end sometime, so we have to savour every morsel."

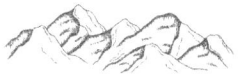

Date:_____

"Life is like a good meal. We know it's going to end sometime, so we have to savour every morsel."

Date:_____

"Life is like a good meal. We know it's going to end sometime, so we have to savour every morsel."

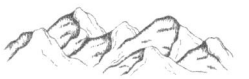

Date:_____

"Life is like a good meal. We know it's going to end sometime, so we have to savour every morsel."

Date:_____

"Life is like a good meal. We know it's going to end sometime, so we have to savour every morsel."

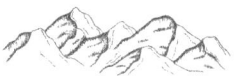

Date:_____

"Sometimes we need inspiration as a reminder to perspire."

Date:_____

"Sometimes we need inspiration as a reminder to perspire."

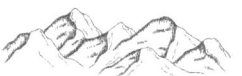

Date:_____

"Sometimes we need inspiration as a reminder to perspire."

Date:_____

"Sometimes we need inspiration as a reminder to perspire."

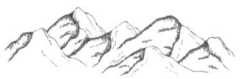

Date:_____

"Sometimes we need inspiration as a reminder to perspire."

Date:_____

"Sometimes we need inspiration as a reminder to perspire."

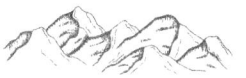

Date:_____

"Sometimes we need inspiration as a reminder to perspire."

Date:_____

"Sometimes we need inspiration as a reminder to perspire."

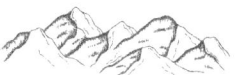

Date:_____

"Sometimes we need inspiration as a reminder to perspire."

Date:_____

"Sometimes we need inspiration as a reminder to perspire."

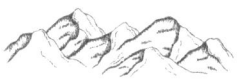

Date:_____

"Sometimes we need inspiration as a reminder to perspire."

Date:_____

"Sometimes we need inspiration as a reminder to perspire."

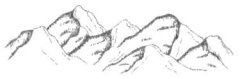

Date:_____

"Sometimes we need inspiration as a reminder to perspire."

Date:_____

"Sometimes we need inspiration as a reminder to perspire."

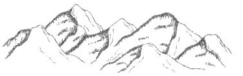

Date:_____

"Sometimes we need inspiration as a reminder to perspire."

Date:_____

"Sometimes we need inspiration as a reminder to perspire."

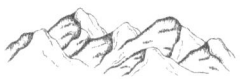

Date:_____

"Sometimes we need inspiration as a reminder to perspire."

Date:_____

"Sometimes we need inspiration as a reminder to perspire."

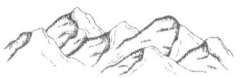

Date:_____

"Sometimes we need inspiration as a reminder to perspire."

Date:_____

"Sometimes we need inspiration as a reminder to perspire."

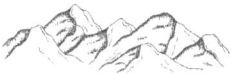

Date:_____

"Sometimes we need inspiration as a reminder to perspire."

Date:_____

"Sometimes we need inspiration as a reminder to perspire."

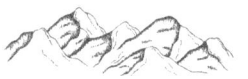

Date:_____

"Sometimes we need inspiration as a reminder to perspire."

Date:_____

"Sometimes we need inspiration as a reminder to perspire."

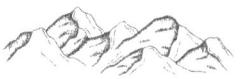

Date:_____

"Sometimes we need inspiration as a reminder to perspire."

Date:_____

"Sometimes we need inspiration as a reminder to perspire."

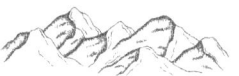

Date:_____

"Sometimes we need inspiration as a reminder to perspire."

Date:_____

"Sometimes we need inspiration as a reminder to perspire."

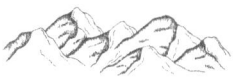

Date:_____

"Sometimes we need inspiration as a reminder to perspire."

Date:_____

"Sometimes we need inspiration as a reminder to perspire."

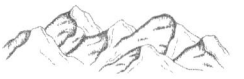

Date:_____

"Challenges are like building blocks. Each one we experience strengthens us."

Date:_____

"Challenges are like building blocks. Each one we experience strengthens us."

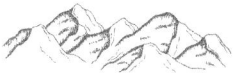

Date:_____

"Challenges are like building blocks. Each one we experience strengthens us."

Date:_____

"Challenges are like building blocks. Each one we experience strengthens us."

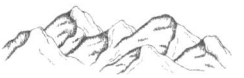

Date:_____

"Challenges are like building blocks. Each one we experience strengthens us."

Date:_____

"Challenges are like building blocks. Each one we experience strengthens us."

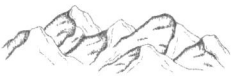

Date:_____

"Challenges are like building blocks. Each one we experience strengthens us."

Date:_____

"Challenges are like building blocks. Each one we experience strengthens us."

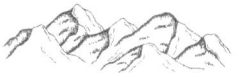

Date:_____

"Challenges are like building blocks. Each one we experience strengthens us."

Date:_____

"Challenges are like building blocks. Each one we experience strengthens us."

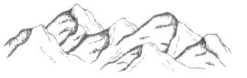

Date:_____

"Challenges are like building blocks. Each one we experience strengthens us."

Date:_____

"Challenges are like building blocks. Each one we experience strengthens us."

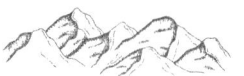

Date:_____

"Challenges are like building blocks. Each one we experience strengthens us."

Date:_____

"Challenges are like building blocks. Each one we experience strengthens us."

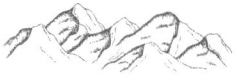

Date:_____

"Challenges are like building blocks. Each one we experience strengthens us."

Date:_____

"Challenges are like building blocks. Each one we experience strengthens us."

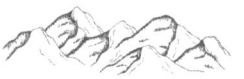

Date:_____

"Challenges are like building blocks. Each one we experience strengthens us."

Date:_____

"Challenges are like building blocks. Each one we experience strengthens us."

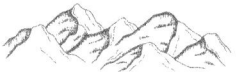

Date:_____

"Challenges are like building blocks. Each one we experience strengthens us."

Date:_____

"Challenges are like building blocks. Each one we experience strengthens us."

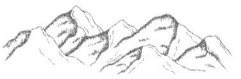

Date:_____

"Challenges are like building blocks. Each one we experience strengthens us."

Date:_____

"Challenges are like building blocks. Each one we experience strengthens us."

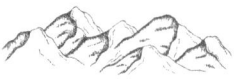

Date:_____

"Challenges are like building blocks. Each one we experience strengthens us."

Date:_____

"Challenges are like building blocks. Each one we experience strengthens us."

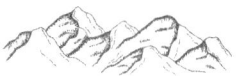

Date:_____

"Challenges are like building blocks. Each one we experience strengthens us."

Date:_____

"Challenges are like building blocks. Each one we experience strengthens us."

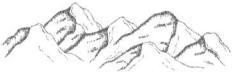

Date:_____

"Challenges are like building blocks. Each one we experience strengthens us."

Date:_____

"Challenges are like building blocks. Each one we experience strengthens us."

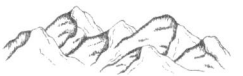

Date:_____

"Challenges are like building blocks. Each one we experience strengthens us."

Date:_____

"Challenges are like building blocks. Each one we experience strengthens us."

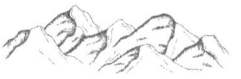

Date:_____

"At the end of the day, the complete body of work, not individual gains and losses, measures success."

Date:_____

"At the end of the day, the complete body of work, not individual gains and losses, measures success."

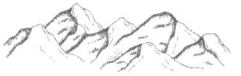

Date:_____

"At the end of the day, the complete body of work, not individual gains and losses, measures success."

Date:_____

"At the end of the day, the complete body of work, not individual gains and losses, measures success."

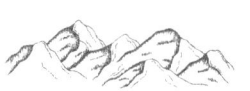

Date:_____

"At the end of the day, the complete body of work, not individual gains and losses, measures success."

Date:_____

"At the end of the day, the complete body of work, not individual gains and losses, measures success."

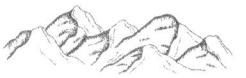

Date:_____

"At the end of the day, the complete body of work, not individual gains and losses, measures success."

Date:_____

"At the end of the day, the complete body of work, not individual gains and losses, measures success."

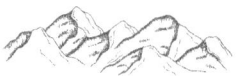

Date:_____

"At the end of the day, the complete body of work, not individual gains and losses, measures success."

Date:_____

"At the end of the day, the complete body of work, not individual gains and losses, measures success."

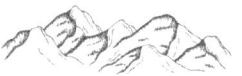

Date:_____

"At the end of the day, the complete body of work, not individual gains and losses, measures success."

Date:_____

"At the end of the day, the complete body of work, not individual gains and losses, measures success."

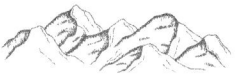

Date:_____

"At the end of the day, the complete body of work, not individual gains and losses, measures success."

Date:_____

"At the end of the day, the complete body of work, not individual gains and losses, measures success."

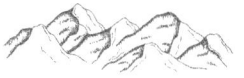

Date:_____

"At the end of the day, the complete body of work, not individual gains and losses, measures success."

Date:_____

"At the end of the day, the complete body of work, not individual gains and losses, measures success."

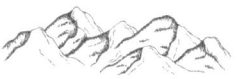

Date:_____

"At the end of the day, the complete body of work, not individual gains and losses, measures success."

Date:_____

"At the end of the day, the complete body of work, not individual gains and losses, measures success."

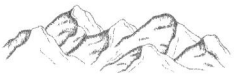

Date:_____

"At the end of the day, the complete body of work, not individual gains and losses, measures success."

Date:_____

"At the end of the day, the complete body of work, not individual gains and losses, measures success."

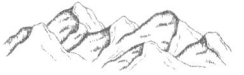

Date:_____

"At the end of the day, the complete body of work, not individual gains and losses, measures success."

Date:_____

"At the end of the day, the complete body of work, not individual gains and losses, measures success."

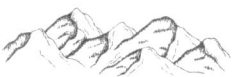

Date:_____

"At the end of the day, the complete body of work, not individual gains and losses, measures success."

Date:_____

"At the end of the day, the complete body of work, not individual gains and losses, measures success."

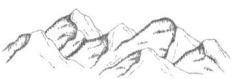

Date:_____

"At the end of the day, the complete body of work, not individual gains and losses, measures success."

Date:_____

"At the end of the day, the complete body of work, not individual gains and losses, measures success."

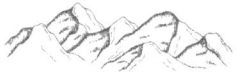

Date:_____

"At the end of the day, the complete body of work, not individual gains and losses, measures success."

Date:_____

"At the end of the day, the complete body of work, not individual gains and losses, measures success."

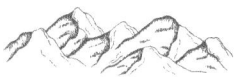

Date:_____

"At the end of the day, the complete body of work, not individual gains and losses, measures success."

Date:_____

"At the end of the day, the complete body of work, not individual gains and losses, measures success."

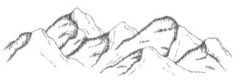

Date:_____

"Every mountain top is within reach if you just keep climbing."

Date:_____

"Every mountain top is within reach if you just keep climbing."

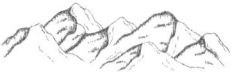

Date:_____

"Every mountain top is within reach if you just keep climbing."

Date:_____

"Every mountain top is within reach if you just keep climbing."

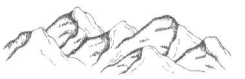

Date:_____

"Every mountain top is within reach if you just keep climbing."

Date:_____

"Every mountain top is within reach if you just keep climbing."

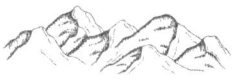

Date:_____

"Every mountain top is within reach if you just keep climbing."

Date:_____

"Every mountain top is within reach if you just keep climbing."

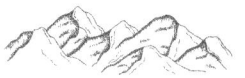

Date:_____

"Every mountain top is within reach if you just keep climbing."

Date:_____

"Every mountain top is within reach if you just keep climbing."

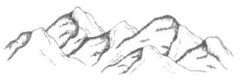

Date:_____

"Every mountain top is within reach if you just keep climbing."

Date:_____

"Every mountain top is within reach if you just keep climbing."

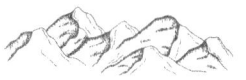

Date:_____

"Every mountain top is within reach if you just keep climbing."

Date:_____

"Every mountain top is within reach if you just keep climbing."

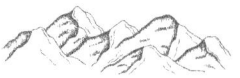

Date:_____

"Every mountain top is within reach if you just keep climbing."

Date:_____

"Every mountain top is within reach if you just keep climbing."

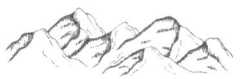

Date:_____

"Every mountain top is within reach if you just keep climbing."

Date:_____

"Every mountain top is within reach if you just keep climbing."

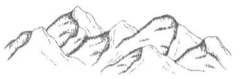

Date:_____

"Every mountain top is within reach if you just keep climbing."

Date:_____

"Every mountain top is within reach if you just keep climbing."

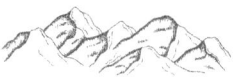

Date:_____

"Every mountain top is within reach if you just keep climbing."

Date:_____

"Every mountain top is within reach if you just keep climbing."

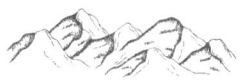

Date:_____

"Every mountain top is within reach if you just keep climbing."

Date:_____

"Every mountain top is within reach if you just keep climbing."

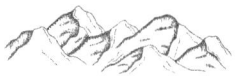

Date:_____

"Every mountain top is within reach if you just keep climbing."

Date:_____

"Every mountain top is within reach if you just keep climbing."

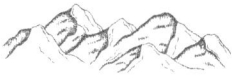

Date:_____

"Every mountain top is within reach if you just keep climbing."

Date:_____

"Every mountain top is within reach if you just keep climbing."

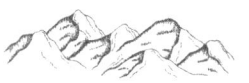

Date:_____

"Every mountain top is within reach if you just keep climbing."

Date:_____

"Every mountain top is within reach if you just keep climbing."

www.ingramcontent.com/pod-product-compliance
Lightning Source LLC
Chambersburg PA
CBHW051547010526
44118CB00022B/2605